Naturopathic Herbal Remedies

For Kids

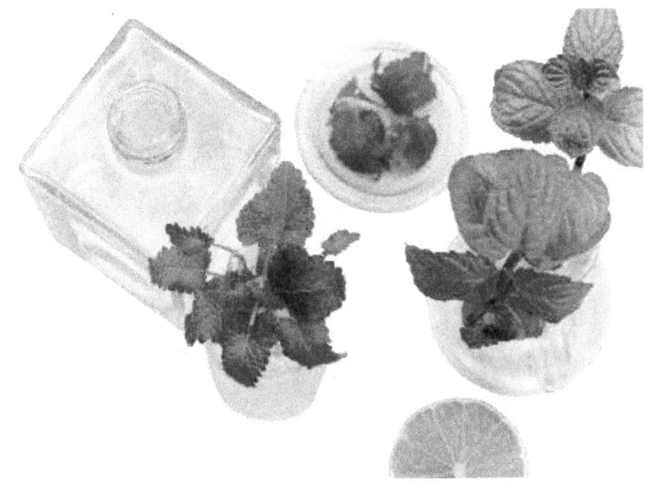

Simple and Delightful Quests for the Young at Heart

Kristie J. Morrison

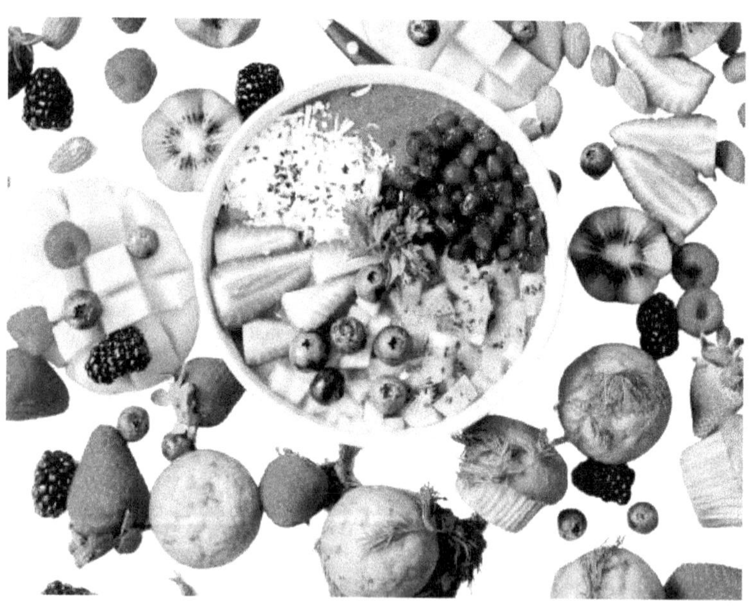

Table of Contents

INTRODUCTION

Young Toby's curiosity ignited in a sun-kissed hamlet. However, his chronic cough hindered his daily activities. Then fate brought him to a magical book, whose pages whispered Echinacea and Thyme secrets. Toby, armed with optimism, wandered the fields and woods, seeking therapeutic plants. As the sun coated the sky with gold, Toby sat by the window, holding his teacup. The herbal infusion, warm and aromatic, swirled in the beautiful porcelain.

With each drink, the cough that had been bothering him for days faded, like a reserved guest exiting a party too early. The room seemed to be holding its breath, waiting for the magic to happen. And then, at that silent moment, Toby exhaled—a long, uninterrupted breath. His chest stopped trembling, and the raspy echoes were replaced by quiet.

The herbal tea's warmth filled him, expelling darkness. Toby's popularity spread; he was a boy who danced with nature's force, demonstrating that believing can cure.

In the gentle embrace of nature's wealth, a world of healing and wonder awaits children's inquisitive minds. "Naturopathic Herbal Remedies for Kids" is more than a book; it is a voyage into the heart of well-being, where each leaf and root tells a story of health and energy.

This is a book that translates the earth's whispers and harnesses the power of plants to nourish the body, boost the spirit, and inspire the imagination. Herbal treatments are an old interaction between people and the natural world, one that has fostered our species from time immemorial.

Herbal treatments constitute an ancient dialogue between people and the natural world, one that has nourished our species since time immemorial. These cures are the product of many years of wisdom that recognizes our deep connection to the plant kingdom. As I embark on this journey, I offer children the opportunity to participate in this time-honored tradition by exploring the benefits of herbal treatments through enjoyable and healthy excursions that are both informative and entertaining. Each chapter in this book is a step forward in learning how basic herbs can be transformed into powerful health friends.

By explaining their benefits, demystifying their preparation, and enjoying making them, I will explain what it means to use herbal remedies. From the sunny meadows where chamomile blossoms to the kitchen where a pot of echinacea tea simmers, we will travel together, learning and smiling along the way.

I open the entrance to this lush realm with caution and respect. Safety is the compass that guides our exploration, ensuring that the excursions I take are not only enjoyable but also safe. This book will provide clear directions and safeguards, allowing parents and children to use herbal treatments safely and confidently.

"Naturopathic Herbal Remedies for Kids" is an invitation to a world where health is an adventure, every remedy is a treasure to be discovered, and the knowledge of the earth is the greatest gift we can give our children.

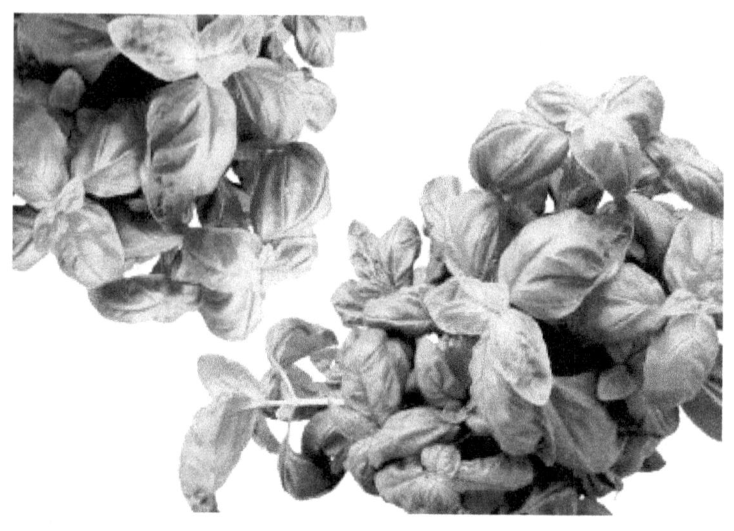

CHAPTER 1

The Green Foundation

Children from a nearby community met at "The Green Foundation," a beautiful garden, to learn about plants' healing properties. Sage, the knowledgeable owl, directed them to Aloe Vera, Minty the Mint Plant, and Lavender, each with unique medical benefits.

Sage taught children to respect and care for these herbal friends, emphasizing the importance of adult supervision and conservation. Inspired, the children created the Herbal Adventure Diary to document their findings and experiences. This garden was a starting point for learning about nature's medicines, sparking a lifelong path of research and respect for the natural world.

Understanding Herbal Remedies

Imagine having a little green friend who loves to pamper you when you're sick. This friend is not a doctor, but a plant from your garden. Herbal remedies are like special secrets that plants share with us to help us feel better.

They are made from different parts of plants, like leaves, flowers, or roots, and each part has its own superpower to help with things like a tummy ache or a scrape on your knee.

The History and Philosophy of Herbal Medicine

Long ago, even before doctors, people discovered that plants might help them heal. They saw animals eating specific plants when they were sick, and they learned from them.They eventually started using these plants to heal themselves. The theory, or big idea, of herbal medicine is that nature has provided us with everything we require to be well and happy. It is like having a treasure box in your backyard filled with natural delicacies that can make you feel happy.

The Role of Herbs in Modern Naturopathy

Today, we have something called naturopathy, which acts as a treasure map, guiding us to natural ways to stay healthy. Natural herbs are included in this map because they guide us to optimal health, like a compass.

Naturopathy teaches us that by employing herbs and other natural ingredients, we may help our bodies heal themselves, similar to how superheroes heal after saving the day.

Decoding the Language of Plants

Plants cannot communicate like humans, but they do have their own language. If we pay attention, we can grasp what they are saying. Some plants, for example, have bright, colorful flowers that may be saying, "Hey, I can help make you feel more cheerful!" Other plants emit powerful odors that can say, "I will help clear up your stuffy nose!".

Decoding plant language means determining what their colors, shapes, and fragrances are attempting to convey about how they might help us feel better.

Lily and the secret language of plants:

In "The Secret Language of Plants," a wise tree teaches young Lily how plants communicate through their leaves and blooms. She learns that:

- Bright green leaves indicate a cheerful and healthy plant.
- Yellow or brown leaves may suggest the need for additional maintenance.
- Blooming flowers indicate a healthy plant; however, drooping blossoms indicate a problem.

As Lily develops into a plant whisperer, she assists her green friends, who repay her in their quiet manner.

Fun Plant Fact: Did you know that bamboo can grow nearly a meter (3.2 feet) in just one day? This plant is faster than any other in the world. So, if plants could speak, bamboo would probably remark, "I am the fastest one in the plant kingdom!"

CHAPTER 2

The Herbal Pantry

The herbal pantry is a hidden gem in the corner of every healer's kitchen, where jars of dried herbs and bottles of infused oils stand in neat rows like wise old sage. Each herb, from the soothing chamomile to the energizing peppermint, contains a story and a solution within its leaves and flowers.

This pantry offers more than just storage; it is a gateway to well-being, where youngsters may learn about natural treatments. They learn how to make tea for a peaceful night's sleep, salves for skinned knees, and potions to lift their spirits.

It is a location where the traditional wisdom of naturopathy meets the inquisitive minds of youth, producing a legacy of health and natural harmony.

Preparing Your First Remedies

Hello, tiny healers! Are you prepared to produce your first herbal remedies? It is like being a culinary scientist. You might begin with something simple, such as a relaxing tea.

Simply choose a soothing herb, such as chamomile for relaxation or peppermint for a pleasant stomach, and immerse it in hot water. It is just like giving your herbs a warm bath. With adult help, filter the leaves and make a therapeutic tea.

Herbal Tea Infusion

Ingredients:

- 1-2 tablespoons dried chamomile flowers
- 1 cup boiled water.

Instructions:

- Put the chamomile flowers in a cup and cover with boiling water.
- Cover and steep for 5 to 10 minutes.

- Strain and consume before bedtime for a calming effect.

Turning Herbs into Healing Brews

Turning herbs into therapeutic brews is a lot of fun. Assume you are creating a potion that grants superpowers. Use fresh or dried herbs and soak in water. This is referred to as steeping, and the herbs appear to be giving the water all of their secrets. After they have talked for a while, you will get a magical drink that can make you feel better or give you extra energy.

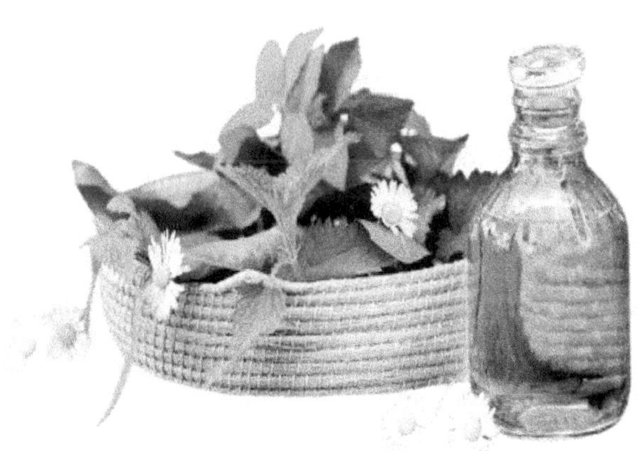

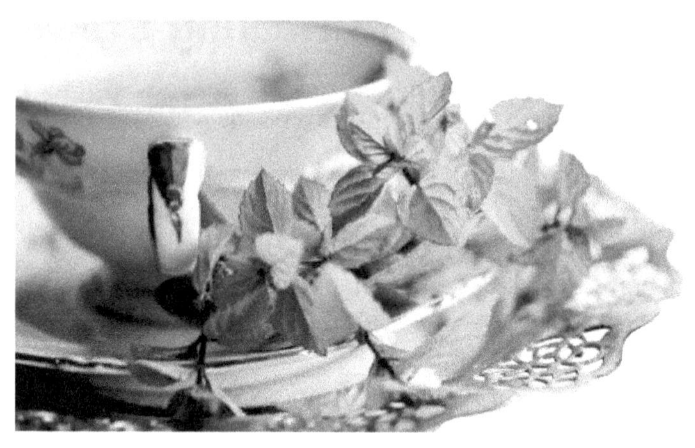

HEALING BREWS

The Art of Infusions, Ointments, and Syrups

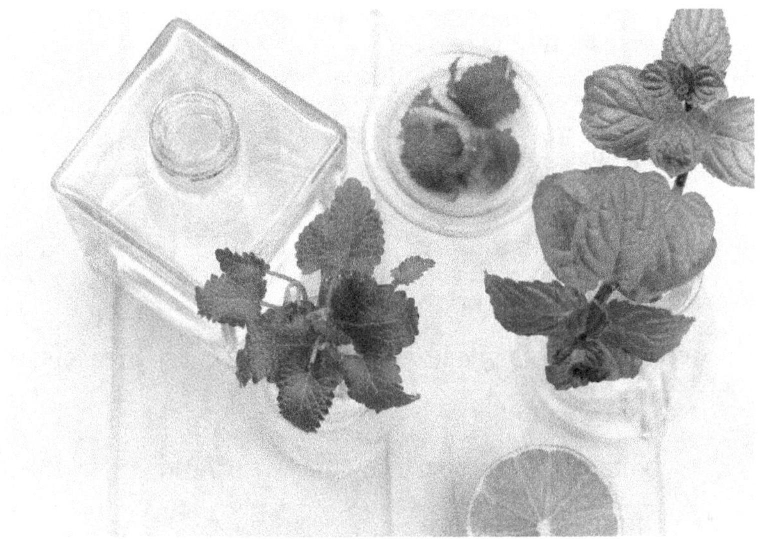

Infusions are like herb superheroes trapped in little drops. It is mixed with something powerful, such as vinegar or glycerin, and left for several weeks. To take the infusion, use a dropper with adult supervision.

Mint Infusion

Ingredients:

- Fresh mint leaves
- vinegar or glycerin.

Instructions:

- Fill a container with fresh mint leaves and cover with vinegar or glycerin.
- Seal the jar and keep it in a cool, dry area out of direct sunlight.
- Shake the jar every few days and allow it to steep for 6 to 8 weeks.
- Strain the infusion through cheesecloth and store it in amber glass bottles.

Ointments are creamy creams that are massaged onto the skin. They are mixed with beeswax and oil to make a silky balm for scratches or dry skin.

Ingredients:

- Half a cup of beeswax (this will give your salve the proper texture).

- A few drops of lavender essential oil (for a lovely scent and an added relaxing effect).
- 1 cup of olive or coconut oil (both soft on the skin).
- Half a cup of dried calendula petals (excellent for calming the skin).

Instructions:

- **Infuse the Oil:** In a jar, combine the olive oil and calendula petals.
- **Allow to marinate**: Close the cover and leave it in a sunny area for a week. This allows all the benefits of the flowers to be absorbed into the oil.
- **Strain the Petals**: After one week, remove the petals with a sieve, leaving only the infused oil.
- **Melt the beeswax**: Melt the beeswax in a double boiler (one saucepan filled with water and another bowl on top). Take care; it is hot! This should be done by an adult.
- **Mix everything.** Once the beeswax has melted, mix in the infused oil.
- **Add the scent:** Turn off the heat and add a few drops of lavender essential oil for a delightful aroma.

- **Pour into the container:** Pour the mixture carefully into small jars or tins and allow it to cool. Once it has cooled, it will be solid and ready to use.
- **Label your ointment**: Make a fun label for your ointment so you can remember what it is and when it was made.

There you have it! Your homemade ointment can treat minor scrapes or dry skin.

Safety Tip: Remember to have an adult assist with the heating sections and enjoy your natural creation.

Syrups are created by boiling herbs with a lot of sugar or honey. They are ideal for relieving sore throats or simply as a tasty treat. Remember, little ones, always have an adult present when making these medicines, and only use herbs that are safe for children. Have fun exploring and creating.

Ginger Honey Syrup.

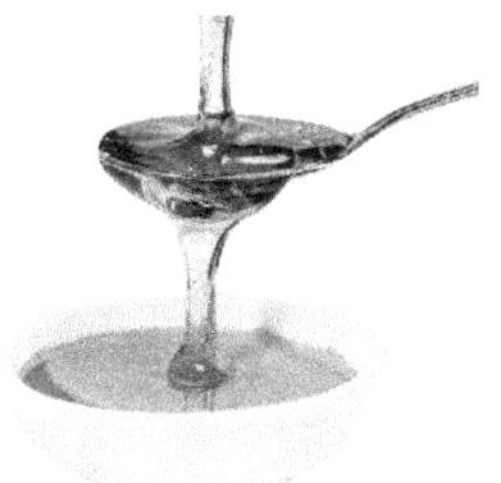

Ingredients:

- 1 cup of honey
- Thinly sliced fresh ginger root
- 1 cup of water.

Instructions:

- Bring a pot of water and ginger to a boil.
- Reduce the heat and let the liquid simmer until it has been reduced by half.
- Strain the ginger pieces, then combine the leftover liquid with honey.
- Refrigerate in a glass jar, then use a tablespoon to help digestion or relieve a sore throat.

Fun plant fact:

Chamomile

- Picture tiny fairies sipping chamomile tea in floral glasses.
- Chamomile is like a warm blanket for your stomach, comforting you when you feel like a cranky dragon.

Mint:

- The mint plant emits subtle murmurs. When you rub their leaves, they laugh and say, "Cool down, little adventurer."
- Mint is the superhero of fresh breath, like a minty knight protecting your mouth fortress.

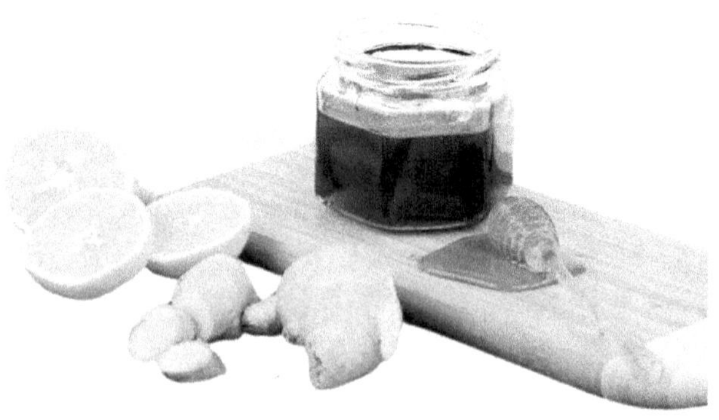

Safety First

Guidelines for Preparing and Using Herbal Remedies

1. **Adult supervision**: Children should never create herbal remedies without an adult present to assist them and ensure they are following the right processes.

2. **Know Your Herbs**: Make certain that the herbs you're using are healthy for children. Some herbs are too strong for young children; therefore, it's crucial to use gentle, child-friendly herbs.

3. **Clean Hands and Surfaces**: Before starting, wash your hands and make sure the surfaces and utensils are clean to avoid spreading germs.

4. **Avoid Touching Your Face**: While handling herbs, children should avoid touching their eyes, nose, and mouth to prevent discomfort or the spread of germs.

5. **Use the Correct Amount**: Because herbs are potent, they must be used in the proper amounts. Follow the recipe or instructions exactly.

6. **Be Aware of Allergies**: If a child has allergies, especially to plants or pollen, make sure the herbs won't cause an allergic reaction.

7. **No Tasting Unknown Plants**: Children should never taste or eat any plant material unless an adult confirms it's safe to consume.

8. **Keep Herbs Away from Pets**: Some herbs can be harmful to pets, so keep all plant materials out of reach of family animals.

9. **Label Everything**: All homemade herbal items should be clearly labeled with the contents and the date they were made.

10. **Store properly**: Keep herbal treatments in a safe area, away from direct sunlight, heat, and dampness, and out of reach of younger siblings.

CHAPTER 3

Garden Adventures

The Garden Adventures is a chapter in which the backyard transforms into a world of discovery and enchantment for children. As they approach their gardens, they are met by a chorus of aromatic herbs and whispering leaves, each enticing them on a different trip.

Here, kids learn to listen to stories of plants, from bold basil, which repels pests, to wise rosemary, which remembers everything.

With their hands in the soil and the sun on their backs, the children transform into intrepid herbalists on a journey to discover the secrets of nature's pharmacy, creating potions and treatments to bridge the gap between the green world and their own. It is a growth chapter for young plants and the adventurers who nurture them.

Growing and Harvesting Herbs

Take the delightful path of herb production and collection. It all starts with selecting the ideal location (a sunny site with well-drained soil) and looking for herbs that are appropriate for the climate's culinary needs. Each herb, from the brilliant green of basil to the delicate fronds of dill, contributes something distinct to the landscape. As your herbs mature.

Learn the Art of Harvesting: Snipping leaves just above a leaf node stimulates bushier growth while gathering blooms and seeds at their optimal flavor.

Planting Seeds of Health: Let us make a small garden. Use a tiny pot or a backyard nook. Sprinkle the seeds lightly into the soil, cover with a layer of dirt, and water thoroughly.Talk to them, sing to them, and soon you'll see little green shoots appear to say hello. It's like having a lot of little green playmates.

The Harvest Cycle: Herbs love to grow, and there is a specific time to harvest them. When they are awakened from their sleep and the sun begins to shine, they are ready to be harvested. Use your fingers to carefully pinch off the leaves; remember not to take too much so that the plant may continue to grow. It is like giving your herb plant a beautiful cut.

Project: Little Green Thumbs: Our Herb Adventure

Materials needed

- A small garden plot or planting containers
- potting soil
- Plant markers.
- Herb seeds (basil, parsley, oregano, and mint are excellent starters).
- A watering can
- Paint and brushes are used to decorate pots.

Instructions:

- **Decorate Your Pots:** Before you start planting, make your pots look amazing. Grab your paints and brushes, and let your creativity run wild.Paint pots with tiny bugs, rainbows, or even your favorite animals. Once completed, let them dry in the sun.

- **Planting Seeds:** Fill the pots with potting soil, leaving a little space at the top. It's time to plant the seeds. Create a small hole in the earth with your finger, insert a seed, and carefully cover it. Remember, seeds are like little treasures that must be tucked into beds under a nice covering of earth.

- **Water Wonders:** Water your seeds with only enough water to moisten the soil, like a damp sponge. Don't use too much, or you'll create a puddle party that the seeds will dislike.

- **Sunlight and Song:** Place your pots where they will receive lots of sunlight. Plants enjoy spending time in the sun. And if you sing to them, they might grow quicker. All excellent gardeners know this hidden trick.

- **Watch them grow:** Give your plants some water every day, and watch them expand and grow. The first shoots will appear in no time. It is like watching a slow-motion race to the top.

- **Harvest Time:** When your herbs have grown large and strong, it is time to harvest them. Pick the leaves gently; they can be used to prepare great dinners. Consider using your home-grown basil on a pizza.

- **Cook for a Day:** Now comes the greatest part! For your family, prepare a dinner with your collected herbs. You may prepare mint lemonade or herb-infused spaghetti. It is a delicious reward for all of your hard work.

- **Plant Party:** Don't forget to have a plant party. Invite your friends to see your herb garden. You can even give them a small plant or seed to take home. Sharing is caring, after all.

- **The Green Guardian:** Your task as a green guardian is not done. Keep caring for your herbs. Water them, give them plenty of sun, and keep them away from annoying critters. Your herbs will continue to flourish, and you'll have a green friend for life.

Fun plant fact:

Basil:

- Basil leaves are like tiny green kites. When the wind blows, they flutter and whisper, "Pesto Power."
- Adding basil to spaghetti enhances its flavor and creates a satisfying meal.

Rosemary

- Rosemary sprigs like tiny wizards with scented wands. They exclaim, "Abracadabra memory boost."
- You can remember where you put your secret treasure map with rosemary.

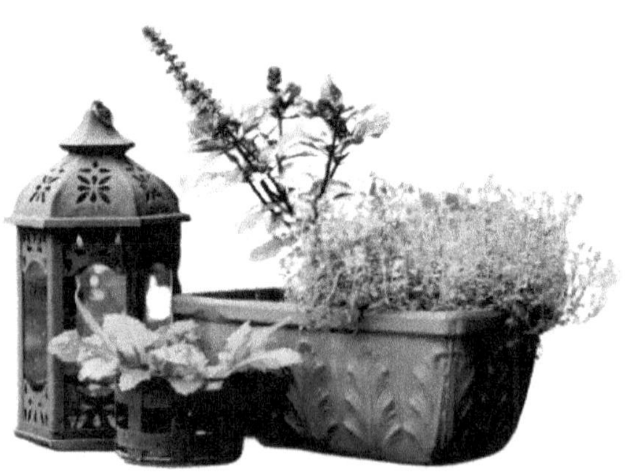

Fun Projects

Making Herbal Soaps and Bath Bombs

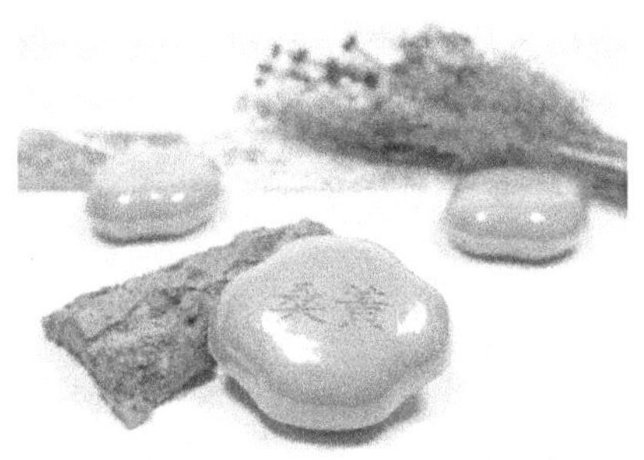

Now, for some fun! With the herbs you have harvested, make soapy concoctions and bubbly bath bombs. Mix the herbs with soap to make it smell nice, or add them to a bath bomb mixture to watch it foam and bubble in the tub.

Herbal soap for kids is a fun and natural way to clean.

Ingredients:

- 10 drops of essential oil (such as lavender or chamomile).
- 1/4 cup dried lavender or chamomile buds.
- 1 kilogram of unscented glycerin soap base.
- Silicone molds with fascinating shapes

Instructions:

- **Prepare the herbs**: Using chamomile, crush the buds slightly to release the smell. Lavender buds can be left entire for a more textured appearance.
- **Melt the soap**: Cut the glycerin soap base into small cubes and heat in a double boiler or microwave in short bursts, stirring regularly, until liquid.
- **Add the herbs**: Once the soap base has melted, add the dried chamomile or lavender buds.
- **Scent Your Soap:** Add the essential oil to the melted soap base, stirring carefully to mix.
- **Pour into molds:** Carefully transfer the soap mixture to the silicone molds. Tap the molds carefully to get rid of any air bubbles.
- **Set the Soap**: Allow the soap to cool and harden for several hours, or until fully set.
- **Unmolding**: Unmold the soaps by gently popping them out of the molds.
- **Cure**: Allow the soaps to cure on a rack for a few days to ensure they are gentle on your skin.

Safety Tips:

- Always supervise children during the soap-making process, especially when melting the soap base and working with essential oils.
- Ensure that the herbs and essential oils used are not sensitive to children's skin.

And now, after making our herbal soap, it is like being a wizard in the world of scents and bubbles. And, guess what? These wonderful masterpieces make ideal, heartfelt gifts for friends and family.

Miniature gardeners and craftsmen! These steps, from the dirt to the tub, have provided hours of pleasure with herbs.

Fun plant fact:

Lavender

- Close your eyes and picture a field of purple and lavender. The air smells of dreams and sleepy clouds.
- Lavender is a sensory lullaby that sings, "Sweet dreams, little stardust."

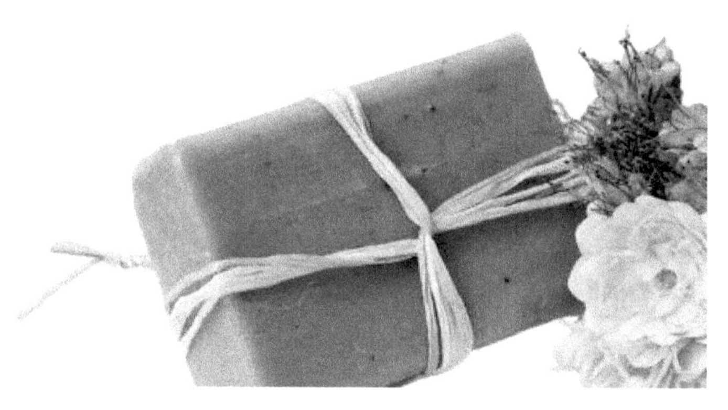

HERBAL SOAP

CHAPTER 4

The Herbalists' Playbook

Welcome to the world of herbal delights, where every leaf and petal is an invitation to adventure! Here are some basic, but fun, activities and experiments for you to try:

Potion Brewing: With the guidance of an adult, create an amazing herbal drink. Combine peppermint for a refreshing zing, chamomile for a relaxing effect, and lemon balm for a burst of sunlight.

Plant a seed. Experience the thrill of producing your own herbs. Start with something simple, such as basil or parsley. Plant the seeds in a pot, water them, and watch them grow every day.

Herbal Art: Create natural artwork using leaves and flowers. To create stunning designs, either press them onto paper or use their juices to paint a masterpiece.

Kitchen Lab: Making a DIY herbal ointment can transform your kitchen into a science lab.

- **Skin cure:** To soothe the skin, combine beeswax, coconut oil, and your preferred dried herb, such as calendula.

Crafting herbal storybooks

Learning Through Tales: Consider the possibility that the garden's plants could communicate stories. What tales would they tell? It's possible to write a storybook about the adventures of brave leaves and intelligent flowers. Pick herbs, learn their names and particular qualities, and then write and draw their epic travels with a vivid imagination. Perhaps the mint leaf can save the day with its fresh breath, or the lavender flower might sing lullabies to let everyone sleep peacefully.

"The Song of Chamomile Meadow"

In Whispering Valley, Lily found a beautiful chamomile patch. Each flower contains a secret: inhale its aroma, and a fantasy will develop. Lily flew across sun-drenched fields, touched the sky, and shared her fantasies with others. Cammy, the chamomile keeper, disclosed her ancient purpose: to absorb hope from human dreams.

Lily pledged to promote compassion by spreading chamomile seeds everywhere. The whispers of chamomile spread optimism over the valley, weaving magic into hearts.

"The Berry Brigade's Quest"

Berry the Strawberry, Bramble the Blackberry, and Minty the Blueberry embark on a daring adventure deep in the Berry Wood Forest. What is their goal? Locate the mythical elderberry, whose purple fruit possessed restorative powers beyond description.

They marched through dense vines and moss-covered glades. Bramble's thorns kept them safe, while Minty's laughter kept spirits up. Finally, they arrived at the Elderberry Grove. The old tree rustled its leaves, revealing bunches of succulent fruit. Berry, Bramble, and Minty filled their baskets. Back at home, they created a wonderful elixir.

Sick villagers drank it; their symptoms dissipated like dawn mist. As a result, the Berry Brigade became heroes, their berry-filled hearts overflowing with pride.

"The Lavender Lullaby"

Young Oliver couldn't sleep in Meadow Brook, a lovely community. His mind worked like a beehive, pursuing anxieties and fears. One beautiful night, Grandma Elsie tucked him in, her eyes gleaming. "Listen, my dear," she murmured, putting a sachet of dried lavender beneath his pillow. As the aroma engulfed Oliver, he dropped off into dreams. The lavender fairies danced and whispered calming charms. His fears dissipated like dewdrops on flowers. Oliver then slept easily, surrounded by Lavender's embrace. And every night, Grandma Elsie sang the most beautiful lullaby, her voice conveying the beauty of flowering meadows.

The Herbal Scavenger Hunt

A Quest for Plant Knowledge: Put on your explorer hats; we are going on a scavenger quest. Our objective is to find as many diverse herbs and plants as possible. Take a peek in your garden, at the park, or along a nature trail.

Can you see a daisy, a pine cone, or a feather? How about a leaf shaped like a heart? Remember to look carefully, and you will discover a secret world of plants all around you.

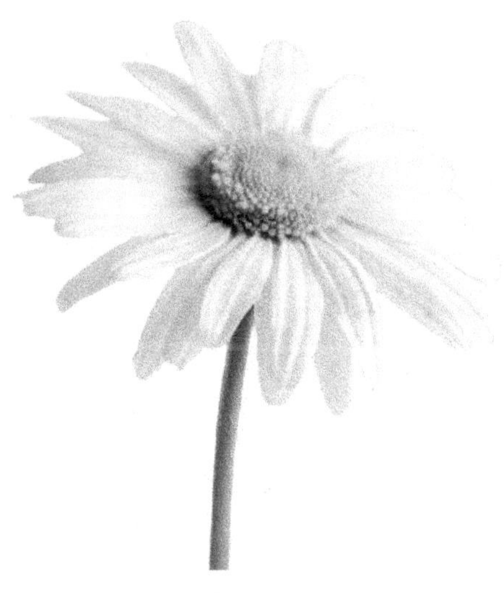

Herb Scavenger Hunt: Make a list of common herbs and see how many you can find in your garden or nearby park. Remember to take notes on their colors, fragrances, and where you got them.

Wholesome Herbal Snacks for Energetic Explorers

After all that sightseeing and storytelling, you must be hungry. Allow us to prepare some energy-packed snacks that will keep you satisfied. What about some oatmeal energy balls with raisins and cinnamon? Or how about some herbal popcorn dusted with rosemary and thyme? These snacks are more than simply yummy; they are like small energy boosters that allow you to run faster, leap higher, and play longer.

Herbal Popcorn

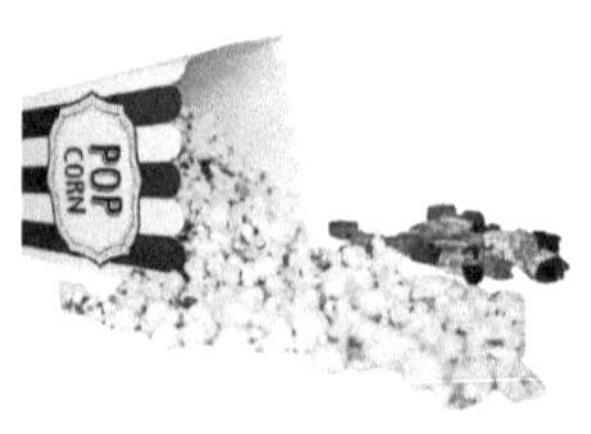

Ingredients:

- Half cup popcorn kernels.
- 1 teaspoon of dried rosemary.
- 1 tablespoon of unsalted butter melted.
- 1 teaspoon of dried thyme
- To taste, add salt.
- 2 tablespoons of vegetable oil (or any high-temperature oil).

Instructions:

- **Pop the corn**: Warm the oil in a big pot over medium heat. Cover the popcorn kernels with a lid. When the kernels start to pop, gently shake the pot back and forth over the flame. When the popping stops, turn off the heat.
- **Prepare the herbs**: While the popcorn is popping, crush the dried rosemary and thyme in a small bowl. This helps to release their flavors.
- **Mix It Up**: Pour the melted butter over the popped corn. Sprinkle crushed herbs on top, along with a

sprinkle of salt. Put the cover back on the saucepan and shake it to evenly coat the popcorn.

- **Taste and Serve:** Give your herbal popcorn a taste, and add additional salt if needed. Serve it in a large bowl so everyone can share!

Safety Tip: Always have an adult assist with the stove and hot oil. To avoid burns, use oven mitts when shaking the pot.

Easy No-Bake Oatmeal Energy Balls with Cinnamon

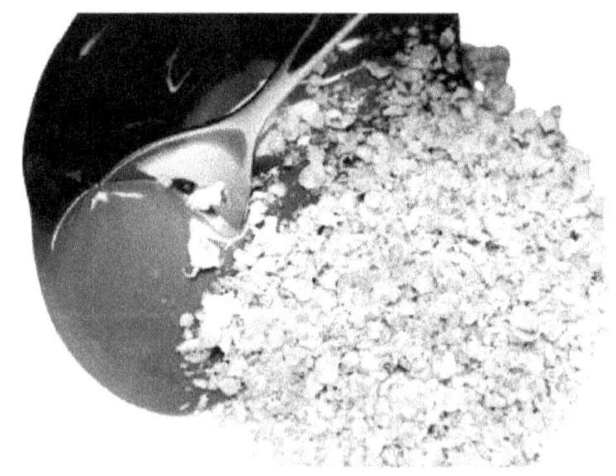

Ingredients:

- 1 teaspoon of ground cinnamon
- 1 cup of old-fashioned oatmeal
- A quarter cup of honey
- 1/2 cup almond butter (or any butter of your choice)
- Optional ingredients include small chocolate chips, raisins, chopped nuts, or dried fruit.

Instructions:

- In a mixing bowl, add oats, almond butter, honey, and ground cinnamon.
- Mix thoroughly until all components are uniformly distributed.
- If desired, include all your favorite mix-ins (small chocolate chips, raisins, or chopped nuts) and mix again.
- Roll the mixture into small balls (about 1 tablespoon each).
- Place the energy balls on a parchment-lined tray or dish.
- Refrigerate for at least 30 minutes until firm.
- Enjoy it as a nutritious snack.

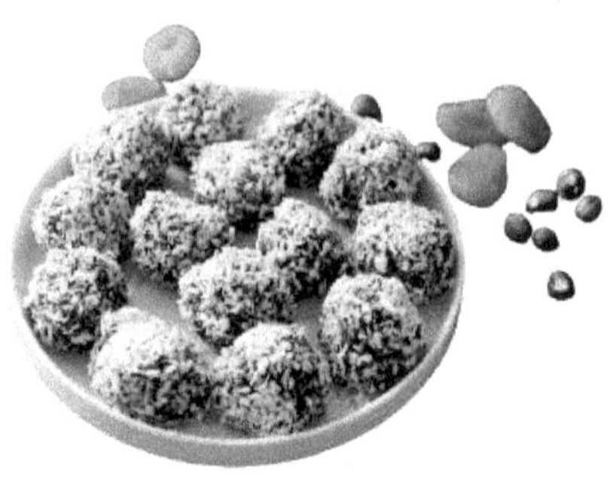

Fun Activities and Healthy Recipes

Hey, kids, are you ready to become a kitchen wizard? Let's make some satisfying snacks that are fun to make and eat. Try preparing a tasty smoothie or a crunchy trail mix with nuts and seeds. A funny face salad with a variety of bright vegetables can be made. Cooking can be a fun game when tasty, healthful delicacies are mixed, matched, and created.

Nutty Berry Blast Smoothie

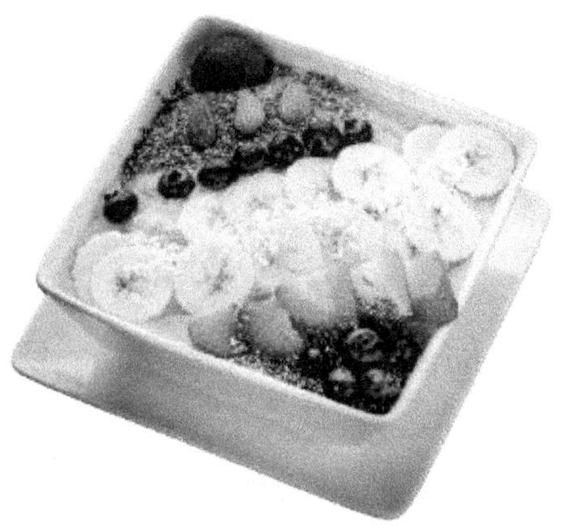

Ingredients:

- 1 tbsp mixed seeds (chia, flax, and pumpkin seeds)
- One ripe banana
- 1 cup fresh or frozen mixed berries (such as strawberries, blueberries, and raspberries)
- 1 tablespoon honey (or to taste)
- Crush 2 tablespoons of mixed nuts (almonds, walnuts, and cashews).
- A quarter cup of plain Greek yogurt
- Half a cup of milk (any sort will work)

Instructions:

- **Prepare the Ingredients**: If using fresh berries, properly clean them. Peel and chop the banana into bits. Crush the nuts into little pieces, but not too fine; it is enjoyable to discover little nutty gems in your smoothie.
- **Blend the base:** In a blender, add the berries, banana, honey, Greek yogurt, and milk. Blend until smooth.
- **Add Crunch:** Combine the crushed nuts and seeds in the blender. Give it a brief pulse to blend them into the smoothie while keeping the crunch.
- **Taste Test**: Have a little taste. If you believe it needs additional sweetness, add a bit more honey.
- **Serve:** Pour your smoothie into glasses and enjoy. If desired, you can sprinkle a few more seeds on top for decoration.

Fun Plant Fact:

Elderberries

- Elderberries are little purple gems fairies use to create sparkling potions.

- Elderberry syrup acts as a superhero shield for your immunity.

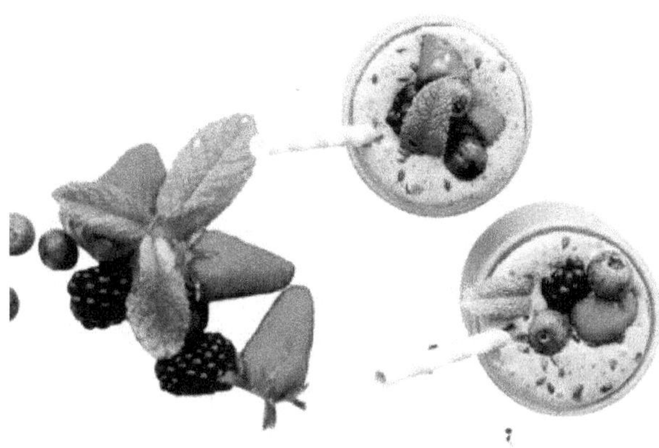

Beyond The Book

Continuing Education in Herbal Remedies: Consider learning about herbal medicines as a never-ending treasure hunt. There is always something fresh to uncover. Continue learning about herbs, like in school. You can start with peppermint tea, then lavender pillows. The more you study, the more you can achieve.

The Herbal Diary

Documenting Your Adventures: Keeping an herbal adventure diary is similar to being a ship captain and writing down all of the wonderful things you discover on your journeys. Draw pictures of the plants you're using, write out how you produced your medicine, and even stick in some leaves or petals. It is a fun opportunity to reflect on all your trips and see how much you've learned.

CHAPTER 5

The Journey Continues

Building a Lifetime of Herbal Wisdom

Building a lifetime of herbal wisdom is like creating a beautiful garden in your head. For each new herb you learn, consider planting a seed in this garden. Perhaps one day you will learn how to create a relaxing chamomile tea and plant a chamomile seed.

Another day, you discover that lavender might help you sleep, so you plant a lavender seed beside it. Your garden will grow with all kinds of plants, each with a secret to making you and your friends feel better as you learn more.

Just as a real garden requires water and sunlight to thrive, so too does your herbal wisdom garden. You might share your herbal secrets with others, such as a garden bouquet.

They can implement these concepts in their gardens, and before long, everyone will have a lovely, flowering garden of herbal wisdom. So, remember that every little amount you learn adds up, and before you know it, you will have a lifetime of herbal knowledge to enjoy and share. Like a garden, it will grow if you nurture it.

Passing the torch

Sharing Herbal Traditions with Friends and Family: Sharing herbal traditions is similar to handing down family recipes. You can teach your friends how to brew a calming chamomile tea or show your family how to produce plants. It is a wonderful way to care for the people you love and help them learn.

MY HERBAL DIARY

My Herbal Journey Begins

Date Started:

Why I Love Herbs:

Write a few sentences about what excites you most about learning and using herbs

My Herbal Discoveries

Herb Name::
____

Discovery Date:
____

What I learnt:

Share interesting facts or uses of herbs you explored
____
____
____
____
____
____

My Experience:

Describe what you did with the plant and how it went
____
____
____
____
____
____
____
____

My Herbal Creations

Creation Name: _Name of Remedy_

Creation Date:

Ingredients Used:
List the herbs and other ingredients you used

Steps Taken:
Outline the process you followed to make your creation

Tell us how your creation turned out and what you learned from it

My Herbal Garden

Planting Date:

Herbs Planted:

List the herbs you have planted in your gardens or pots

Growth Observations:

Note any changes or growth you see in your herbs

Herbal Recipes I Have Tried

Recipe Name :
____

Cooking Date:
____

Ingredients and Steps:
Write down the recipe and steps you followed
____
____
____
____
____
____
____
____
____
____

Taste Test:
Share your thoughts on how the recipe turned out
____
____
____
____
____

Herbal Remedies I Have Used

Remedy Name :

Use Date:

Purpose
Explain why you used this remedy and for what condition.

Effectiveness:
Reflect on how effective the remedy was and how it made you feel.

My Herbal Questions & Answers

Question: *Your Question*
____

Answer: *What you found out*
____
____
____

Date Answered:
____
____

Sources for Answer:
____
____
____
____
____
____
____
____
____

Final Thoughts

As your herbal adventures continue, use this space to write down any final thoughts, future plans, or the dreams you have for your journey with herbs.

Sketches and photos

This is a space for you to draw your favorite herbs or paste pictures of your herbal projects and creations.

Sketches and photos

This is a space for you to draw your favorite herbs or paste pictures of your herbal projects and creations.

Sketches and photos

This is a space for you to draw your favorite herbs or paste pictures of your herbal projects and creations.

Sketches and photos

This is a space for you to draw your favorite herbs or paste pictures of your herbal projects and creations.

Sketches and photos

This is a space for you to draw your favorite herbs & paste pictures of your herbal projects and creations.

Sketches and photos
This is a space for you to draw your favorite herbs or paste
pictures of your herbal projects and creations

Sketches and photos

This is a space for you to draw your favorite herbs or paste pictures of your herbal projects and creations.

This is a space for you to draw your favorite herbs or paste pictures of your herbal projects and creations.

Sketches and photos

This is a space for you to draw your favorite herbs or paste pictures of your herbal projects and creations.